THE
MERCK
INDEX

☆

TWELFTH EDITION
ON CD-ROM
VERSION 12:1
1996

for Microsoft® Windows™

USER GUIDE

D0339081

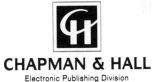

CHAPMAN & HALL
Electronic Publishing Division
London · Weinheim · New York · Tokyo · Melbourne · Madras

Published by Chapman & Hall, 2–6 Boundary Row, London SE1 8HN

Chapman & Hall, 2–6 Boundary Row, London SE1 8HN, UK

Chapman & Hall GmbH, Pappelallee 3, 69469 Weinheim, Germany

Chapman & Hall USA, 115 Fifth Avenue, New York, NY 10003, USA

Chapman & Hall Japan, ITP-Japan, Kyowa Building, 3F, 2-2-1 Hirakawacho, Chiyoda-ku, Tokyo 102, Japan

Chapman & Hall Australia, 102 Dodds Street, South Melbourne, Victoria 3205, Australia

Chapman & Hall India, R. Seshadri, 32 Second Main Road, CIT East, Madras 600 035, India

CD-ROM

ISSN 1359-2947

User Guide

Written by Janet E. Ash

First edition 1996

© 1996 Chapman & Hall

Printed in Great Britain by George Over Ltd, Rugby

TECHNICAL SUPPORT

For support on installation or use of the programs:

Technical Support Desk
Electronic Publishing Division
Chapman & Hall
2-6 Boundary Row
London SE1 8HN   UK

Tel: +44 (0)171 410 6929
Tel: 1 888 306-5235 *in the USA and Canada (toll free)*
Fax: +44 (0)171 522 0101
E-mail: tech.support@chall.co.uk

The Technical Support Desk is open during office hours from Monday to Friday. At other times an answerphone will operate.

If your query concerns your system set-up rather than problems with searching the database, please be prepared to supply the following information to the Technical Support Desk staff when you call:

- description of the problem, including any error messages displayed
- make and model of PC, including size of RAM and hard disc
- make and model of CD drive
- version of operating system and MSCDEX
- contents of CONFIG.SYS, AUTOEXEC.BAT, SYSTEM.INI and WIN.INI files
- display driver details from Windows Setup in the Main program group

For data queries (information in the Monographs):

Ann Smith
Associate Editor, The Merck Index
Merck & Co., Inc
P.O. Box 2000
Rahway NJ 07065, USA

Tel: +1 (908) 594-6310
Fax: +1 (908) 594-1187
e-mail: ann_smith@merck.com

JOIN US ON THE INTERNET

WWW: http://www.thomson.com
EMAIL: findit@kiosk.thomson.com

A service of I(T)P®

CONTENTS

INTRODUCTION

Chapman and Hall and Merck & Co., Inc., have joined forces to produce *The Merck Index on CD-ROM*, which contains the monograph section of the 12th edition of *The Merck Index* and selected tables. The database includes more than 10,000 monographs, each describing a single substance or small group of related compounds. It covers human and veterinary drugs, biologicals, natural products, agricultural compounds, commercial and laboratory chemicals and environmentally significant compounds. The CD-ROM contains powerful text and substructure searching software for exploring the contents of the database.

Software for installation and use of the database is provided on the CD-ROM. For details of the hardware and software requirements, and the installation instructions see the inside of the front cover of this manual.

The programs used for searching the database are:

- Headfast/CD from Head Software International for searching, retrieving and displaying the text, structure diagram and data associated with each compound.

- PsiBase for Windows from Hampden Data Services, for searching, retrieving and displaying chemical structures.

The text and structure searching modules are linked with a seamless interface, so that you can move from text to structure searching, and vice versa, without being aware of having changed from one system to another. Both modules operate under Microsoft Windows™ Version 3.1 or Windows 95, hereafter referred to as Windows.

You do not need to have any experience with online searching, or with the use of CD-ROM products, but some knowledge of the Windows operating environment is assumed.

A sample guided search for new users is given on page 3.

Not all of the options available for searching the CD-ROM are given in this short manual. Further details of the options are given in the electronic Help screens.

The integration of structure and text allows you to:

- use the structure search facilities to refine the results of a text search.

- display the text associated with a compound retrieved as a result of a structure search.

- use the text search facilities to refine the results of a structure search.

An explanation of all the icons used as buttons on the text searching and the structure searching screens is given on pages 46-51.

For more details about the database, the contents of the searchable fields, and abbreviations used in the database consult the electronic Help screens.

SAMPLE GUIDED SEARCH

The following is an example of a text search followed by structure search.

SEARCH QUERY: Find all compounds which are used as an antiseptic, then see which of those compounds are chlorinated aromatics.

Starting to use The Merck Index on CD-ROM

Double click on The Merck Index icon to display the main menu.

Click on **Quick Search** (the simplest level of text searching) to display the list of fields you can search.

Click on **All Text**, which will enable you to find all entries which contain the word ANTISEPTIC. You can now enter the search term using the Index, or by typing the search term directly into the Search box at the bottom of the screen.

Using the index to enter search terms

When you first open the index, the cursor is positioned in the Index Stem box. The letter A is already in the Index Stem box. Continue to type the word:

ANTISEPTIC

As you type, the index will move down to the entry which is nearest alphabetically to the one you have typed. When you see the word ANTISEPTIC in the index, double click on it to transfer the word to the Search Term box at the bottom of the screen. If you make a mistake, click on the dustbin button (**Clear Terms**) in the button bar at the top of the screen.

You will see that the word ANTISEPTICS also occurs in the index, so you must also enter this as a search term. Double click on the word ANTISEPTICS in the index to transfer that term to the Search Term box. The "/" symbol, which represents OR, is automatically inserted between the search terms.

N.B. Although the "/" is added automatically, you must insert any other search relation required when entering search terms, e.g. AND and NOT. All the possible search relations are given in the Operator Toolbox, which is displayed when you click on the **Toolbox** icon:

Entering the search terms without using the index

You can also enter the search terms without using the index. When you click on the **All Text** field, the index is displayed, but you can type the search term directly into the Search Term box. Position the cursor in the Search term box at the bottom of the screen and click the mouse.

Type the search term:

ANTISEPTIC*

You should use the wildcard * at the end of the word so that ANTISEPTIC and ANTISEPTICS will be retrieved.

Searching the database

Click on the **Search** icon in the tool bar to start the search:

Displaying the search results

The summary list of results, showing about 190 hits, is displayed on the screen, listing the names of the compounds which satisfy the search query. The names are given in Monograph Number order, and thus appear in alphabetical order. You can also display the CAS Registry Number or the Molecular Formula, using the options in the **Format** menu, and you can change the order of the display using the options in the **Sequence** menu.

Click on the up or down arrow buttons to scroll up or down the list of hits, or use the cursor keys. To display the full details about an entry, highlight that entry, then press [**Enter**] or click on the **View Entry** icon:

You can change the display of the full entry, using the options in the **Format** menu. All of the options include the Monograph Number and Title of the compound. If the entry is too long to fit on the screen, click on the arrow button at the bottom right-hand side of the screen to move down the entry.

To superimpose the structure on the screen, click on **Show Diagrams** in the **Options** menu, or click on the **Diagram On/Off** icon (the fifth button in the row). N.B. If there is no diagram available, this option will not be active. You can Move or Close the diagram window, if it is obscuring the text.

To view the full details about the other hits, click on one of the arrow buttons in the toolbar. You can also press [**Enter**] to display the next entry in the hit list.

Before you can carry out the structure search, click on the **Close Entry** icon in the tool bar (the first icon in the row), to go back to the summary display.

Structure Search

With the summary list of hits displayed, click on the **Refine with Structure Search** icon in the tool bar:

The structure drawing screen is then displayed. The structure corresponding to the highlighted entry in the summary display is shown in the middle of the screen. As we are now going to search for chlorinated aromatic compounds, it is easier to clear this structure then draw the required structure from a clear screen.

To clear the structure, click on the **File** menu, then click on **New**, or click on the **New Structure** icon in the toolbar:

The structure drawing tools are shown on the left-hand side of the screen, and the Pencil Tool, at the top, is highlighted. This is used for drawing and modifying individual atoms and bonds.

Drawing the structure

To draw the simplest substructure to represent chlorinated aromatic compounds, draw 3 aromatic ring atoms, then attach a chlorine atom to the middle one.

Start by drawing a chain of 3 carbon atoms as follows:

Click on the Chain Tool (the third tool in the drawing palette). A dialog box is displayed giving a default chain length of 1. Press the backspace key, then type in the number 3. Click on **OK**. The cursor changes to a chain. Position the cursor in the center of the screen and click the mouse to draw a 3-carbon chain.

To draw the chlorine atom attached to the middle of the 3-carbon chain, click on the Pencil Tool (the cursor changes to a pencil). You must now change the Current Atom at the bottom of the screen to a chlorine atom. Click on **Cl** in the atom/bond palette. Position the point of the cursor over the center carbon atom in the chain*, then press and hold the mouse button down whilst you drag the cursor away from the atom to form a new bond. Release the mouse button and a chlorine atom will be drawn attached to the center carbon atom.

*You will see a little **A** appear in the middle of the pencil cursor, when the cursor is correctly positioned over an atom.

If you make a mistake when structure drawing, you can:

1.   Clear the drawing screen completely: click on **File**, then **New**.

2.   Delete the last action: click on **Edit**, followed by **Undo**.

3.   Click on the Eraser Tool, immediately below the Chain Tool. To erase an atom, position the end of the eraser over the atom, then click the mouse. To erase a bond, position the end of the eraser over the center of the bond, then click.

Query definition

When you have drawn the structure, you must define the specific attributes required when you use the structure as a query. You must therefore define the carbon-carbon bonds to be aromatic before you carry out the search. Otherwise, you will retrieve any structure that has a chlorine atom attached to a carbon chain.

6

Before using the Query definition options, you must select the bonds. Click on the Selection Tool (immediately below the Eraser Tool), and the cursor changes to a box shape.

Position the cursor over the center of one of the carbon-carbon chain bonds, and click the mouse button to highlight the bond. Then hold down the Shift key and position the cursor over the other carbon-carbon chain bond and click. If you do not hold down the shift key, you can select only one bond.

Click on the **QueryDef** menu, then click on **Bond Characteristics**. Click on **Ring** under Bond Type and click on **Normalized** under Bond Value.

Query verification

You must now verify that you have defined the correct attributes for the atoms and the bonds. Click on the **QueryDef** menu again, then click on **Query Verification**. Click on **OK** to verify all the rings, nodes and bonds. Each type of bond, node and ring will be highlighted in turn, where appropriate, and details of the attributes are given at the bottom of the screen. You should have two normalized ring bonds, three ring nodes (the carbon atoms), one chain atom (the Cl atom) and one chain bond. Click on OK each time to move on to the next box. If you have made any mistakes, go back to the query definition again.

Searching

Click on the **Search** menu, then on **Preferences**. Click on **Continuous** under View hits, and **Yes** under Prompt (these may already be selected). Click on the box next to **Use Previous Results** (unless there is already a cross "×" in the box). Make sure there is no cross in the box next to **Exact Search**. If there is a cross, click on the box to remove it.

Click on **OK**.

Click on the Search menu, then on **Start** to display the initial search box. **Use Text Results** means that the search will be carried out on the results of the text search.

Click on **Continue** to start the screening search (a fast search of the database to select possible candidates for detailed search). The number of hits from the screen search is displayed (about 30).

Click on **Continue** to proceed with the atom-by-atom search. The hits are displayed as the search proceeds and then the final number of hits is shown (about 10).

Click on **Continue** again and you will be prompted to enter a name for the results set just created. Then click on **OK**.

Viewing the structure search results

Click on **Search**, followed by **Browse Hits**. A dialog box is displayed. Click on **Continuous**, then on **Next**, to display the hits one after another on the screen, or just click on **Next** to display the next hit. Click on **Cancel** when you wish to stop browsing through the hits.

Alternatively, you can return to the text Summary display to list the hits: click on **Search**, then on **Text Search**. When you have displayed the Summary list, you can view the hits as described in the section on **Displaying the Search Results** on page 4.

To print any of the hits from the summary list, either as a list or as complete entries, select **Print** in the **File** menu, or click on the **Print** icon. You will be prompted to choose between printing the summary list, marked items, unmarked items, or the currently highlighted item. You can mark or unmark items by clicking on the **Mark** icon, or by pressing the **F8** key.

Entries may also be transferred to the clipboard for export, for example to word processing packages. Select the whole text, or part of the text, then click on **Edit**, **Copy**. You can then choose to copy the whole text, the selected part, or just the diagram to the clipboard.

GETTING STARTED

Find the Merck Index icon, and double click to display the introductory screen:

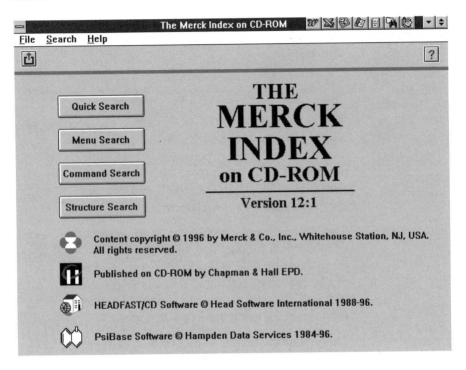

Fig. 1: Main Menu

You can now choose whether to start with a text/data search, or a structure search. If you want to do a text search, you have the choice of:

Quick Search,   Menu Search or Command Search

The three levels of searching are explained on page 10.

To start with a structure search, click on **Structure Search**, and go to page 25 for instructions on structure searching.

TEXT AND DATA SEARCHING

There are three levels of text and data searching:

- Quick Search
- Menu Search
- Command Search

<table>
<tr><td></td><td></td><td align="right">See
page</td></tr>
<tr><td>Quick Search</td><td>This is the simplest level of searching and is used for searching a single field, such as a Trade name, or a particular therapeutic category. You can use more than one search term, linked by AND, OR, NOT, and you can use * to truncate the search terms.</td><td align="right">13</td></tr>
<tr><td>Menu Search</td><td>The menu search enables you to enter a simple search for one field, or to search across more than one field at a time. A selection of 6 of the available searchable fields is displayed and you can add or remove fields from the drop-down list using the + or − sign icons.</td><td align="right">15</td></tr>
<tr><td>Command Search</td><td>This is a more flexible search method than the menu search. You can search any of the 25 fields available, and you can build up complex search strategies using Command Search by combining different fields.</td><td align="right">17</td></tr>
</table>

Combining search terms

Whichever level of search you choose, you can link the search terms using combinations of AND, OR, NOT, and you can use search relations, such as >, < = when you are searching for numerical data.

Use only the following symbols:

        &   to represent AND

        /   to represent OR

        \\   to represent NOT

All the available options and other search relations are in the **Operator Toolbox** accessed by clicking on the **Toolbox** icon:

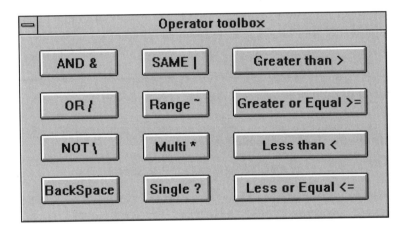

Fig. 2: The Operator Toolbox

Examples of combining search terms are given on the following page.

Special Symbols

The **Special Symbol keypad** contains all the Greek characters and other symbols you may need when entering a search term. You can access this by clicking on the icon:

Truncation and wild cards

Use the following characters as wildcards and for truncation:

* *   to indicate a string of characters – either within the search term, or at either end of the term, to truncate the term

?   to indicate a single letter within a word

You can use a combination of * and ? within a search term.

If you use an * at the end of the search term to truncate the term, it will save entering all the possible variations of the search term. For example, if you search for DISINFECT* in the **Use** field, you will retrieve all compounds which are used as DISINFECTANTS, for DISINFECTING and in DISINFECTION.

Using left hand truncation, you can search for classes of compounds. For example, a search for *OLOL will retrieve all compounds whose names end in OLOL, such as ATENOLOL, LEVOBUNOLOL, PINDOLOL, etc.

Examples of combining search terms

AND

To find all compounds which are both antidepressants and analgesics enter the following search in the **Therapeutic category** field:

ANALGESIC&ANTIDEPRESSANT

OR

To find all compounds which are used as foodstuffs or in animal feed, enter the following truncated search terms in the **Use** field:

FOOD*/FEED*

NOT

To exclude FRUIT or FRUITS from the search this search, enter:

FOOD*/FEED*\FRUIT*

RANGE SEARCH

To search for all compounds with a melting point between minus 5° and plus 8°, enter the following search terms in the **Melting Point** field (Menu or Command Search only):

-5~8

QUICK SEARCH

Use the Quick Search to search for a single word of text, or for a Trade Name, or a CAS Registry number, or a Molecular Formula, for example. You can combine search terms within a given field, using the operators shown on page 11. A sample guided Quick Search is given on page 3.

From the Main menu, click on **Quick Search** to display the list of fields that can be searched.

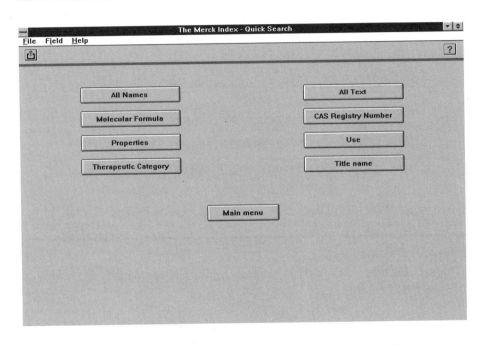

Fig. 3: Quick Search

You can search any of the fields listed. Each field contains an index of all the terms in that field. When you click on a field, the index is displayed for that field. You can enter search terms using the index (see next page), or type the terms directly into the Search Terms box (see page 4), using truncation to enter long chemical names (see previous page). For a description of the content of individual fields, use the electronic Help screens. An explanation of the icons at the top of the screen is given on page 46.

Selecting the Search term using the Index

1. Type the first part of the required search term in the Index Stem box (you may need to press Backspace to remove the first entry, or click on the **Eraser** icon - see below for picture of the icon). The correct part of the index will then be displayed. Continue to type the search term until the required term is displayed in the index. Highlight the required term.

2. With the required search term highlighted, double click the mouse to transfer the search term to the Search Term box at the bottom of the screen. Additional search terms may be added by repeating step 1.

3. If you do not want to add any more search terms, click on the **Search** icon to carry out the search.

the eraser icon – clears index stem

the search icon – initiates the search

the previous screen icon

Go to page 20 for instructions on examining the search results.

Sample Quick Search

To find all entries which relate to diabetes or insulin, enter the following search terms into the **All Text** field:

DIABET*/INSULIN*

This will retrieve compounds which contain any of the words Diabetic, Diabetes, Insulin, Insulins.

MENU SEARCH

Menu searching allows you to search more than one field at a time. From the Main menu, click on **Menu Search** to display a list of six searchable fields. You can add other fields to, change, or remove fields from, this list. A complete list of fields is given on page 18. For a description of what is available in each field, use the electronic Help screens.

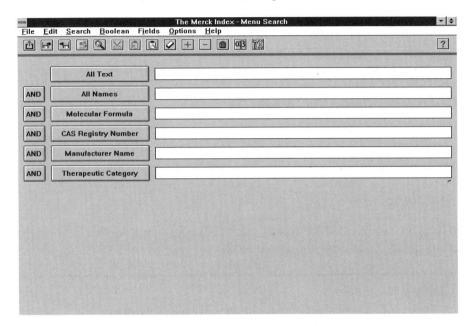

Fig. 4: Menu Search

To enter a search term

Click on the search box adjacent to the required field name. Type in the search term required, or select it from the index (see instructions on page 14).

To display the index, click on the **View Index** icon: [icon]

The meaning of all the other icons on the screen is given on page 47.

You can enter search terms into as many of the search fields as you wish.

To add, delete or change a field in the list of search fields

- **To add a new field**, click on the **+** icon. An All Names field is added to the bottom of the list of fields.
- **To delete a field**, place the cursor in the search box adjacent to the field, and click the mouse, then click on the **–** icon. The field is removed from the list.
- **To change a field**, place the cursor over the button containing the name of the field you want to change, then click the mouse to display the complete list of fields, and click on the required field in the list.

You can save your favorite menu, using the Save option in the File menu.

Linking the fields in the search

You can change the option on the button to the left of the search field. Click on the button to toggle between AND, OR and NOT. You can also combine search terms within a field. Use the Operator Toolbox described on page 11.

Searching

When you have created the search, click on the **Search** icon. See page 20 for instructions on analyzing the search results.

Sample Menu Search

To find all cholesterol-lowering compounds produced by Merck & Co., Inc., change the All Text field to Manufacturer Name, then enter the search terms as follows:

	Manufacturer Name	MERCK*
AND	All Names	
AND	Molecular Formula	
AND	CAS Registry Number	
AND	Use	
AND	Therapeutic Category	ANTIHYPERCHOLESTEROLEMIC/ ANTIHYPERLIPIDEMIC

COMMAND SEARCH

With the Command Search, you can build up a complex search strategy using any of the indexed fields in the database. You can also modify and extend a search, in the light of the results of the first search, and you can store search strategies for future use.

From the Main menu, click on **Command Search**.

The following screen is displayed:

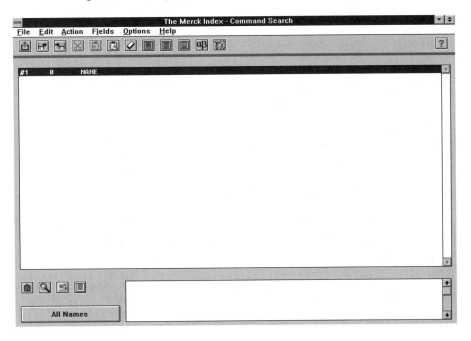

Fig. 5: Command Search

You enter search terms into the search box at the bottom of the screen. The field to be searched is shown in the Field Type box next to the search box. The default is All Names. The main part of the screen gives the search history, with details of all previous searches.

The meaning of all the icons on the screen is given on page 48.

Entering the search term

Before you enter the search term, you must choose the field you wish to search. The list of searchable fields is given in the Fields menu, or is displayed when you click on the button to the left of the Search box (labeled All Names, when you first open the Command Search screen). The searchable fields are shown below:

All Names	Molecular Weight
All Text	Monograph Number
All Entries	Note
Additional Name	Properties
Boiling Point	Refractive Index
CA Name	Rotation
CAS Registry Number	Therapeutic Category
Density	Title Name
Derivative Type	Toxicity
Drug Code	Trade Name
Manufacturer Name	Use
Melting Point	UV Maxima
Molecular Formula	

For a description of the content of each field, use the electronic Help screens.

Click on the Field you wish to search.

N.B. The All Entries field is just a flag, not a searchable field. If you have carried out a search on part of the database, (e.g. the results of a previous search), you can use All Entries to return to searching the whole database. Select **All Entries**, then enter **Y** (yes) as the search term.

When you have selected the field to search, you can then type your search term(s) directly into the search box, or select search terms from the index, as described on page 14. To display the index, click on the View Index icon.

You can add as many search terms as required from the currently selected field, using the operators shown on page 11.

Click on the **Search** icon at the bottom of the screen, or press **Enter** to start the search. The search term is then transferred to the search history box, showing the search query number, the number of hits found, the field type searched and the search term. Each time a search is carried out, the result is stored under the next sequential query number, giving a complete history of all the searches. If you make a mistake, highlight the entry, then click on the **Eraser** icon to clear the entry.

To view the search results, highlight the appropriate line in the Search history box, then click on the **View Results** icon.

Combining searches

You can combine the results of searches. To combine the results of searches 2 and 3, for example, type the following in the Search box:

#2&#3

You can also enter a new search term and combine that with the results of a previous search, for example, the following search request would combine a search for ANALGESIC with the results of search number 4, using OR logic:

ANALGESIC/#4

EXAMINING THE SEARCH RESULTS

When you have carried out a Quick or a Menu Search, the results are displayed as a summary list of hits, giving the names of the compounds. The first compound in the summary list is highlighted. When you carry out a Command Search, you must double click on the required search in the Search History box to display the summary list of hits.

The following icons appear at the top of the summary display:

	Refine search
	Refine with structure search
	Forget text search
	GoTo item
	Print
	Mark/Unmark
	Move to first item in list
	Move up one page
	Move up one item
	View entry
	Move down one item
	Move down one page
	Move to the last entry
	On-screen help

You can go back to refine the text search, or you can proceed to refine the search with a Structure Search.

There are a number of different options for the order and content of the summary list. These options are given in the Format and Sequence menus at the top of the screen:

Format Menu

Name
CAS number and Name
Name and CAS number
Molecular formula and name
Name and Molecular formula

Sequence Menu

By Monograph Number
By CAS Registry number
By Molecular formula

The Sequence menu allows the list of hits to be sorted in ascending order by monograph number, CAS Registry number or molecular formula.

Use the arrow icons to move up and down the list of hits.

You can mark any of the hits, by selecting the hit, then clicking on the **Mark** icon, or pressing F8. A small colored square is displayed to the left of the entry. You can then selectively print the marked entries (or the unmarked ones). To remove the mark, highlight the entry again, then click on the **Mark** icon or press F8 again.

Follow the instructions on the next page to display the full entry.

Displaying and Printing the Entry

To display full details about any of the hits, highlight the required hit, then double click on it, or click on the **View Entry** icon.

You can change the display of the entry using the options in the Format menu:

Option	What is displayed
Book	The complete monograph, as in the printed 12th edition of *The Merck Index*
Full Fielded	The complete monograph, but in a fielded layout with field titles. CAS Registry Numbers are displayed
Compound	Monograph number, title, names of the compound, CAS Registry number, molecular formula, molecular weight and properties
Names and Uses	Monograph number, title, names of the compound, CAS Registry number, trade marks and therapeutic categories
Pharmaceutical	Monograph number, title, CAS Registry number and therapeutic category. Derivatives are also given
Short	Monograph number, title, CAS Registry number, therapeutic category and use.

You can mark the entry by clicking on the **Mark** icon (see page 21 for description of the Mark option).

To display the structure, click on the **Structure** icon. The structure diagram, for the main entry compound, is overlaid on part of the screen. You can move it around by clicking on the title bar and dragging the structure box to the required position. To remove the structure display, click on the **Structure** icon again.

To print the entry currently displayed, click on the **Printer** icon. You must then choose whether you wish to print the text, the structure, or both. You can also copy the entry, or part of the entry, to the Clipboard, using the Edit, Copy option.

LINK TO STRUCTURE SEARCH

If you wish to use a structure search to refine the results of your text search, click on the **Refine with Structure Search** icon:

The structure drawing screen is displayed, showing the structure of the currently highlighted hit from the summary list. You can then browse through the structures of the hits, or refine the results of your text search.

Browsing through the hits

Select the Search menu, followed by List Hits, or Browse Hits.

Refining the results of your text search

Follow the instructions for preparing structure queries in the remainder of this manual.

Then select the **Search** icon:

Click on **Use: Text Results**

The results of the text search will then be used as the search file for the structure search.

STRUCTURE SEARCHING

You can use a structure search on its own, or to refine the results of a text search.

Click on **Structure Search** in the Main Menu to display the structure drawing screen.

To prepare a structure search, you must:

- draw the structure, as described in the section on drawing and editing structures (page 27)
- prepare the structure query, for an exact match or for a sub-structure search, as described in the section on preparing the structure query (page 36).

For further details about all the options in structure searching, consult the electronic Help screens.

The Structure Drawing screen

Click on the Structure Search button in the Main menu to display the Structure Drawing screen:

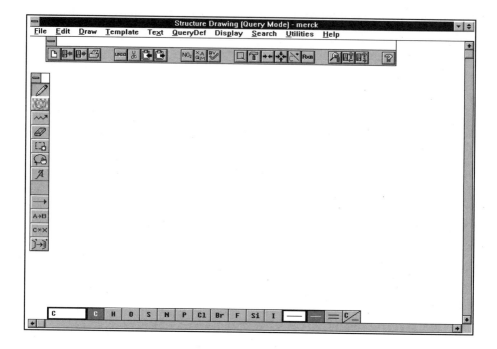

Fig. 6 The Structure Drawing screen

The structure drawing screen consists of:

* a drawing palette containing tools for drawing structures (L.H. side)
* a Common Atoms and Common Bonds palette (bottom of screen)
* a Toolbar (optional) to display buttons for frequently used commands. This can be switched on and off using the Desktop option in the Utilities menu. The icons in the toolbar are explained on page 50.
* a title bar at the top of the screen
* a menu bar with options for drawing, filing, editing, searching and displaying structures

DRAWING STRUCTURES

You can draw structures by:

- using the drawing tools
- calling up a template for editing
- carrying out a text search, then selecting a hit for transfer to "Structure Search", and modifying the structure

The drawing tools

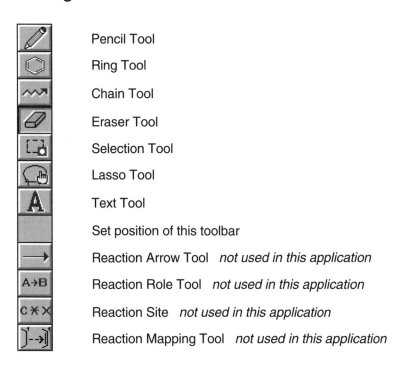

	Pencil Tool
	Ring Tool
	Chain Tool
	Eraser Tool
	Selection Tool
	Lasso Tool
	Text Tool
	Set position of this toolbar
	Reaction Arrow Tool *not used in this application*
	Reaction Role Tool *not used in this application*
	Reaction Site *not used in this application*
	Reaction Mapping Tool *not used in this application*

To draw a structure, use the Pencil Tool, the Ring Tool or the Chain Tool. Select the required tool, then move the cursor to where you want the object, and click the mouse button. The atoms and bonds drawn will be the Current Atom and Current Bond, which shown in black-bordered rectangular boxes at the bottom of the screen. See next section for details of drawing and modifying atoms and bonds.

Pencil Tool

Use the Pencil Tool to draw atoms and bonds. To draw two nodes connected by a bond, position the cursor where you want the first node to be placed. Press and hold the mouse button down, whilst you drag the cursor to the point where you want the second node to appear, then release the mouse button. The atoms and bond drawn will be the Current Atom and Current Bond (see previous section).

Modifying atoms and bonds using the Pencil Tool

Use the Pencil Tool for changing atoms or bonds in the Structure, unless you wish to modify a large number of atoms or bonds, when you should use the Selection Tool.

When the Pencil Tool is correctly positioned over a bond, a small line will appear along the middle of the pencil. Similarly, a small "A" will appear when the pencil is correctly positioned over an atom.

Modifying bonds: If the Current Bond is single, you can draw a double bond by "drawing" another bond over an existing bond: drag the pencil Tool from one node to the other, retracing the existing bond (convert from a double bond to a triple bond in the same way). You can also modify an existing bond by first changing the Current Bond: choose a new bond value from the palette at the bottom of the screen, or from the Bond menu. If you make a single click on the new bond value, it makes a temporary change to the Current Bond (after one use, it reverts to the previous value); whereas a double click on the new bond value makes a permanent change. When you have selected the new bond, place the tip of the cursor on the middle of the bond to be changed and click. The bond will then change to reflect the new Current Bond. (To return the Current Bond to Single, press the Space Bar).

Modifying atoms: First change the Current Atom to the required symbol, by selecting one of the common atoms at the bottom of the screen, or using the Atom menu (again, a single click on the new atom makes a temporary change and a double click makes a permanent change). Place the tip of the pencil cursor over the node to be changed and click. The node will change to reflect the Current Atom. (To return the Current Atom to Carbon, press the space bar.)

Ring Tool

Use the Ring Tool to draw 3- to 15-membered rings. Select the Ring Tool, then type in the ring size, or select one of the pre-defined ring types displayed, and click on **OK**. Position the cursor where you want to draw the ring on the screen, and click. You may continue to use the selected tool to draw similar rings. To draw a spiro ring, position the cursor over an existing ring node and click. The second ring will be spiro fused to the first. To draw a fused ring, position the cursor in the middle of an existing ring bond, and click. The second ring will be fused to the first along the selected bond. Fused ring systems can be drawn using the Feldmann notation, details of which are given in the electronic Help screens.

Chain Tool

Use the Chain Tool to draw chains of length 1 to 30 nodes. Select the Chain Tool, then type in the length of the chain you require. The default is 1. Click on **OK**. Position the cursor where you want the chain to start (either over an existing node, or in a space on the screen) and click. A chain, of the length specified, is drawn in a logical way.

Eraser Tool

Use the Eraser Tool to delete an atom or a bond. Click on the Eraser Tool. To erase an atom, position the tip of the cursor over a node and click. To erase a bond, position the tip of the cursor over the middle of the bond and click.

Selection Tool

Use the Selection Tool to highlight nodes and bonds, before deleting or modifying them, or prior to query definition (see page 36). Click on the Selection Tool and the cursor changes to a rectangle containing a cross. Select items as follows:

a node	position center of cursor over node and click*
a bond	position center of cursor over center of bond and click*
part or all of a structure	draw a rectangle round the structure: position the cursor at the top left hand corner of the rectangle, press and hold the mouse button, then drag the mouse button down across the structure to draw a dotted rectangle encompassing the required group of atoms. Release the mouse button. To deselect one of the selected nodes, position the cursor over the node, press and hold the Shift key and click.

* To select more than one disconnected node or bond, press and hold the Shift key whilst selecting the nodes or bonds.

Lasso Tool

Use the Lasso Tool to select a structure if you want to move it to another location on the screen. When you select the Lasso Tool, the cursor changes to a lasso. Press and hold the mouse button as you drag the cursor round the object to be moved. Release the mouse button, then move the cursor inside the lassoed area. The cursor changes to a hand. Press and hold the mouse button and drag the hand to the new position on the screen. Release the mouse button. To remove the currently drawn lasso, click outside the lasso.

Other tools in the palette

Use of the Text Tool and Reaction Tools are described in the electronic Help screens. Reaction searching is not available on this CD-ROM.

The Draw menu

The Draw menu allows you to select bonds, atoms, shortcut symbols and variable atoms, and to fuse fragments together. Brief details of the use of the Bond, Atom and Shortcut options are given below. For details of the other options, see the electronic Help screens.

Bond

Use the Bond option in the Draw menu to select a new Current Bond value. A box is displayed giving all the possible bond types. Click on the required bond type, then click on **Single Use** or **Multiple Use** according to whether you wish to make a temporary change or a permanent change to the Current Bond.

Atom

Use the atom option in the Draw menu to select a new Current Atom. A box listing all the available atoms is displayed, with the common atoms down the left hand side and the rest of the atoms in alphabetical order. Click on the required atom, then click on **Single Use** or **Multiple Use** according to whether you wish to make a temporary change or a permanent change to the Current Atom. In Query Mode, there is also an option to exclude the selected atom from the search query.

Shortcut

The Shortcuts are predefined common groups of atoms, usually with one point of attachment. You can select a Shortcut in the same way as you select an atom (see above). Some Shortcuts can be drawn in the reverse direction. Click on the small button next to the shortcut, if you want it drawn in reverse.

The Display menu

The options in this menu allow you to change the display of the structure on the screen. Brief details of the options are given in the table below. For further details, see the electronic Help screens.

Carbons	Use this to change the display of carbon atoms from Angle mode to Dot mode or to displaying C symbols
Show VPA	If you have defined an atom with a variable point of attachment, use this option to show all the potential sites of attachment
Show Hydrogens	Displays hydrogens on terminal carbons and heteroatoms with spare valencies
Show Node Numbers	Inserts node numbers on every atom in the structure
Show Reactions	Shows the role, (e.g. reactant, or product) of each compound in the reaction
Smooth	Use this to straighten and align structures that have been drawn freehand
Expand	Enlarges and centers the drawing on the screen
Contract	Contracts and centers the drawing on the screen
Reverse Shortcut	Reverses the display of Shortcut symbols (where available)
Rotate	Rotates a structure about an atom. Pre-select the structure first
Flip fragment horizontal	Use this to flip the structure from left to right or vice versa
Flip fragment vertical	Use this to flip the structure from top to bottom or vice versa
Snap to Grid	Displays a grid on the screen – where possible, bonds are moved to align with the grid lines. To remove the grid lines, click on Preferences in the Utilities menu, then click on Grid
Snap to Compass	Aligns a pre-selected set of nodes to the nearest compass position.

Using Templates: the Template menu

Template files are files of structural fragments, which you may use when drawing your structure. You can add new templates, which contain fragments that you use frequently. You should create a separate sub-directory to contain your own template files.

Open

Click on **Open** to open a template file. A box is displayed giving the list of template files available (or change the directory to locate template files that you have created). Use the mouse to scroll down the list of templates, then click on the template file that you want. The structures in the template will be displayed in the small window. If they are the required structures, click on **Open**.

The fragments in the template file are displayed. Click on a node or bond in the fragment you require, then click on **OK**. You are returned to the drawing window and the cursor changes to a Fusion cursor. Click on a free space to draw the template on its own, or, if you have selected a bond in the template, you can fuse the template structure on to an existing structure by clicking on a bond of the existing structure. For a spiro fusion, you must click on an atom in the template structure and an atom in the existing structure. You will get a warning if the valency of an atom will be exceeded as a result of the fusion.

Edit

Select **Edit** from the Template menu, if you want to modify a template file. Open the required template file, as described above, then you can draw any additional template structures, or editing any of the templates displayed. When you have finished editing the structures, select **Save** to store the structures.

Save

Select **Save** to save the structures currently drawn on the screen as a template. You may change the name of the file in which the templates are stored.

Editing structures: the Edit menu

The Edit menu provides standard editing commands, such as Cut, Copy and Paste. Brief details of the options are given in the table below. For full details, consult the electronic Help screens. Before using the Cut, Copy or Clear commands, you must select the object(s) first in one of the following ways:

- use Select **All** from the Edit menu
- highlight a specific node or bond using the Selection Tool
- use the Selection Tool, or the Lasso Tool, to draw a rectangle or loop round the required atoms and bonds.

Undo	Undo the last action made
Cut	Delete the selected objects and place them on the Clipboard
Copy	Copy selected objects to the Clipboard
Paste	Paste objects from the Clipboard into the current structure drawing window
Select All	Select all the items on the screen
Clear	Delete selected items from the screen
Clear All	Clears the whole screen
Show Clipboard	Display the contents of the Clipboard
Repaint	Update the display on the screen
Delete Mappings	This is not used in this application

Filing and printing structures: the File menu

The File Menu provides commands for opening new and existing files, saving and printing. You can use the options in the File menu to prepare your own structure collections. When preparing structure queries you must use Query Mode. If you just want to draw and print structures, use Structure Mode. Select the **Change Mode** option in the QueryDef menu to change to Structure Mode.

Brief details of the options in the File Menu are given in the table below. For full instructions consult the electronic Help screens.

New	Clear the drawing screen ready to draw a new structure
List File..	Lists all the structures in the currently selected structure collection (indicated in title bar at top of screen). From the list, you can Print, Browse, or Mark structures for deletion.
Browse File	Browse through the structure collection.
Save	Saves structures currently displayed on the screen.
Save As	Saves displayed structure under a new name
Change File	Use this to change the current structure collection
Import	Import structures or queries in other formats.
Export	Export structures in other formats.
Graphics	Creates a file in the PCX format for subsequent use in other Graphics packages
Page Setup	Allows you to set options relating to printing the structure, e.g. page size
Print	Prints the structure currently displayed
Exit	Returns you to the Main text searching part of the application

PREPARING THE STRUCTURE QUERY

When you have drawn the structure query, use the options in the QueryDef menu to define the precise attributes for your query. If you do not define any attributes, the defaults will apply (see page 38).

To set an attribute, you must first pre-select the required node(s), bond(s) or ring, using the Selection Tool, then choose the appropriate command from the QueryDef menu: Ring Isolation, Bond Characteristics, Node Characteristics.

N.B. If you select a mixture of ring nodes, bonds and chain nodes, you will not be able to proceed with query definition.

The QueryDef menu

A summary of the options in the QueryDef menu is given below. For further details consult the electronic Help screens.

Change Mode

To prepare structure queries, you should be in Query Mode (the mode is indicated at the top of the screen). Click on **Change Mode** to change to Structure Mode only if you want to create your own files of structures.

Ring Isolation

This option is active only if you have selected one or more nodes in a ring. Request an Isolated ring if you want the query ring system to exactly match the ring system in the retrieved structures. Choose isolated/embedded if you do not mind if the query structure is embedded within a larger ring system

Bond characteristics

Select one or more bonds of the same type (e.g. all in ring, or all C-C chain bonds). If you select ring bonds, you cannot change the bond type. If you select chain bonds, you can choose whether you want the bonds to occur in a chain, a ring or either when you search. You can choose the Bond value to be Exact, Normalized. Exact/Normalized or Unspecified.

Node characteristics

You cannot change the definition of a ring node. Pre-select a chain node or nodes. You can then choose whether the selected nodes should occur in a chain, or in a ring, or either, when the search is carried out.

Hydrogen Attachments

Use this option to define the number of hydrogen atoms attached to a given node. Pre-select the required node. Under QueryDef click on **Specific** followed by **Exact** or **Minimum** and type in the number.

Non-Hydrogen Attachments

Pre-select a node, then click on **Non-Hydrogen Attachments** to define the number of atoms connected to a given atom.

Other Attributes

To use this command, you must pre-select a node, then you can select **Other Attributes** to change the Charge, Valency or Isotope values on a node.

Delocalized Charge

Pre-select a group of nodes, then select **Delocalized Charge** to specify the required charge over the selected nodes.

Query Verification

When you have defined all the attributes required for your search, click on **Query Verification**, to review the definitions of your query. Click on **All** to view every feature, or click on **Select** then click on the specific features you want to view. Each feature is then displayed in turn, for you to click on **OK**, or **Cancel**. If you cancel at any time, the highlighted nodes or bonds are automatically pre-selected when you return to the editing screen.

Printing out the query structure. Before starting the search, you can print out your query structure together with all the defined attributes. Select the File menu and click on **Print**.

If you just want to print the structure, without listing any attributes, click on **OK**. To list all the attributes you have defined, click on the **Print Attributes** button. Click on the **Print Title** button to print the name of the file in which the query is stored. If you have not stored the query, the print-out will be labeled Untitled.

Query definition defaults

You can carry out a search *without* defining any attributes and the following defaults will apply:

- all nodes and bonds drawn in a chain in the query structure must occur in a chain in the database structure to satisfy the search query
- all nodes and bonds drawn in a ring must occur in a ring
- all rings in the query structure are set to being isolated or embedded (i.e. rings embedded within a larger ring system will be retrieved)
- alternating single and double bonds in an even-membered ring path are normalized
- tautomeric sequences (according to CAS conventions) are normalized
- all bonds in isolated/embedded rings are set to exact/normalized
- bonds between carbon atoms in isolated rings are set to exact
- bonds between heteroatoms (or between a carbon and a heteroatom) in isolated rings are set to exact/normalized
- chain bonds between carbon atoms are set to exact
- chain bonds between heteroatoms or carbon-heteroatom bonds are set to exact/normalized, except the following, which are set to exact

when an oxygen has two bonds to it, neither of which are H, D or T; R–X bonds, where X is a halogen and R is not N, S, Se, Te or O

N.B. The above defaults apply only if you are in Query mode. You can carry out a search if you are in Structure mode, but different defaults apply and you cannot change them.

You can request that rings must be isolated. Chain bond values can be set as Exact or Normalized, or either, or unspecified. Chain nodes can be set as Chain or Ring or either.

SEARCHING THE DATABASE

The Search menu

When you have prepared the search query, and used the options in the QueryDef menu to further define your search, use the commands in the Search menu to carry out the search. First set up the defaults for the search, using the Preferences option in the Search menu, then click on **Start** to initiate the search. The options in the Search menu are described below.

Searching is carried out at two levels:

- an initial screen search (a fragment search of the structure collection)
- an atom-by-atom search of the hits from the screening search

Preferences

Use the Preferences option to set the defaults for the search. The options are given in the following table:

View Hits	Click on **Yes**, to view the hits as they are found
	Click on **No** – the search will proceed without displaying hits
	Click on **Continuous** to display hits continuously
Prompt	Click on **Yes** to be prompted before each stage of the search
	Click on **No** if you want the screen search and atom-by-atom search to proceed without prompts
	Click on **After screen** to be prompted before the atom-by-atom search
Use Screen File in	Fragments used for the screening search are stored on the hard disk in the directory C:\MRCK created during installation
Exact Search	Click on this to carry out an exact structure search
Use Previous Results	Click on this to use the results of the previous search as the search file for the current search

Start

Before starting the search, select the **Preferences** option in the **Search** menu to set the defaults for the Search. Then click on **Start** to display the search dialogue box.

Screen search: The screen search will proceed automatically unless you chose to be prompted at the start of each search phase (using the Preferences option), when you must click on **Continue** to proceed.

Atom-by-atom search: If you have chosen to be prompted before the atom-by-atom search, the number of hits from the screen search will be displayed. Click on **Continue** to proceed with the atom-by-atom search, but you can click on **View Hits**, or **View Continuous** first if you did not set these using the Preferences option. You can also indicate that the search is an Exact Match search, and you can click on **Use Previous Results**. The options selected here will temporarily override your selection in the Preferences option.

To stop the search at any stage, click on **Cancel**.

When the search has finished, the number of hits is displayed.

Click on **Continue** and you are returned to the structure drawing screen. You can then continue to list or browse through the hits, as described on page 42.

List Hits, Browse Hits

The use of these options is described on page 42.

File IDs – not available in this application

Select Hit List

Use this option if you want to perform a structure search on the results from an earlier structure search (in the current search session). A dialogue box is displayed giving a list of the previous results sets and the number of hits obtained. Type in the number of the search required, or click on the required search in the hit list, then click on **OK**.

Combine Hit Lists

You can combine Hit Lists from the current search session, using Boolean operators AND, OR and NOT. To combine searches 1 and 2, type: 1 AND 2. You will be prompted for a name for the new hit list. You must then go back and select the latest Hit list, as described under Select Hit List above.

Save Query

Use this command to store your query. Type the name of the file into the dialogue box. The file will have the extension .STR, but you can overwrite this.

Restore Last Query

Use this command to recall the last query used in searching.

Text Search

When you have finished a structure search, use the Text Search option to proceed with a text search to refine the structure search. If you wish to use a different hit list in the text search, click on **Select Hit List** first.

VIEWING AND PRINTING SEARCH RESULTS

To view the results of the structure search, open the **Search** menu and click on **List Hits** or **Browse Hits** to display the structures of the hits. If you want to display the summary list of hits or the monographs, click on **Text Search**.

List Hits

Click on **List Hits** to display the hit list of structures. You can then Print the hits, Browse through the list, or mark any of the hits for later deletion.

N.B. The Record Number shown preceded by a hash symbol (#) is merely an internal serial number for the structure, and is not related to the Monograph Number.

Browse Hits

Click on **Browse Hits** to browse through the retrieved structures. As each structure is retrieved, a dialogue box is displayed for you to control the direction of browsing. Click on **Continuous** if you want the browsing to proceed through all the hits without intervention. Click on **Edit** to edit the structure currently displayed, and click on **Cancel** to stop browsing.

Printing Hits

If you want to print the hits, click on **List Hits**, then on **Print**. Click on **OK** to print all the structures in your hit list, one per page. You can change the number of structures printed per page, and can print only a marked set of structures or print a given range of hits, by selecting the appropriate options on the dialogue box.

LINK TO TEXT AND DATA SEARCH

You can combine the results of your latest atom-by-atom search with any of the hits lists stored previously (see Combine Hit Lists on page 41), or you can go back to carry out a text search.

Click on **Continue**, then open the Search menu and click on **Text Search**. The summary list of hits from the structure search is displayed. Click on the **File** Menu to display printing options, and the following options for refining searches:

Refine structure search	takes you back to the structure drawing screen to refine the search with another structure search
Refine structure search with text search	gives you the option of a Quick Search, Menu Search, or Command Search
Forget structure search	takes you back to the Text search Main menu

ADDITIONAL FEATURES AVAILABLE IN THE STRUCTURE SEARCHING PROGRAMS

The following features are available within the structure searching programs, but are not described in this manual. Please consult the online Help screens.

- Detailed use of drawing shortcuts
- Drawing fused ring systems
- Adding text to a structure
- Drawing generic structures
- Drawing variable points of attachment
- Drawing repeating groups, square brackets and multipliers
- Different methods of displaying structures, e.g. changing the display of the carbon atoms, showing variable points of attachment, etc.
- Adding structural attributes, such as charges, abnormal valencies

TROUBLESHOOTING

If you are unable to start using the CD-ROM, check the following:

- Is the CD-ROM drive switched on?
- Is the CD inserted the correct way up? (check with your CD-ROM drive manual)
- Is the CD-ROM drive cable connected to the correct port?
- Are both ends of the CD-ROM driver cable secured?
- Are you using the cable that came with the CD-ROM drive?   The cable is not necessarily interchangeable with other cables.
- If your CD-ROM drive uses a controller (interface) card, is it securely seated in the slot?   It may require some pressure to securely fit in place.
- Is the MSCDEX software installed properly?   You may also need to install a device driver into your CONFIG.SYS file. There should be a message to say that MSCDEX has been loaded into memory.
- Is Windows running in 386 Enhanced mode?

COMPACT DISC CARE

You must look after your CD-ROM.

Always:
- Remove from case by holding edges with one hand and depress center-lock with the forefinger of the other hand
- Hold the disc only by the edges
- Clean the disc using a recommended cleaning kit

Never:
- Leave in CD drive overnight
- Bend the disc
- Scratch the surface, or put scotch tape on the disc
- Put near heat
- Clean with solvent, abrasive cleaner, silicon cloth, anti-static sprays, record cleaner

LIST OF ICONS

Quick Search

Icon	Name	Description
	Field Menu	Return to list of fields in quick search menu
	Search	Start the search
	Clear Stem	Clear the Index stem box
	Clear Terms	Clear a term or terms in the search box
	Characters	Special symbol keypad
	Operator Toolbox	Contains tools for combining search terms
		Not available in this application
	Top	Return to the first entry term in the list
	Page Up	Move up the index one page
	Up	Move one term up the index
	Down	Move one term down the index
	Page Down	Move down the index one page
	Bottom	Move to the bottom of the index
	Help	Access to the electronic Help screens

Menu Search

🔼	Main Menu	Return to main menu
	Open	Open a previously saved menu search screen
	Save	Save a menu search screen
	View Index	View index for current field
	Search	Start the search
	Cut	Cut the selected search term and put on clipboard
	Copy	Copy selected search terms to clipboard
	Paste	Insert search terms from the clipboard
	Clear Form	Clear the entire search screen
	Add Slot	Add an extra field to the search screen (max. 9)
	Remove Slot	Remove selected field from search screen
	Clear Slot	Clear current search box
	Characters	Special symbol keypad
	Operator Toolbox	Contains tools for combining search terms
	Help	Access to the electronic Help screens

Command Search

	Main Menu	Return to main menu
	Open	Open a previously saved command search strategy
	Save	Save current search strategy and results
	Cut	Cut the selected search term and put on clipboard
	Copy	Copy selected search terms to clipboard
	Paste	Insert search terms from the clipboard
	Clear Steps	Clear all steps in the search history box
	Add Step	Add a step at the end of the search history box
	Insert Step	Insert a step at the cursor location
	Remove Step	Remove the highlighted step
	Characters	Special symbol keypad
	Operator Toolbox	Contains tools for combining search terms
	Help	Access to the electronic Help screens
	Clear	Clear the term(s) in the Search box
	Search Current Step	Start the search
	View Index	View the index for the current field
	View Results	View the results (you must first highlight the relevant line in the list of results)

Icons at top of summary display

	Refine Search	Return to search screen to refine search
	Refine with Text Search	Refine structure search with a text search (only available after a structure search)
	Refine with Structure Search	Refine text search with a structure search (only available after a text search)
	Forget Text	Ignore text search and return to main menu (only available after a text search)
	Forget Structure	Ignore structure search (only available after a structure search)
	Go To Item	Go to item: you are prompted to enter a number to move up or down a specified number of places
	Print	Prints the summary list or marked, or unmarked, items in the list
	Mark/Unmark	Click on this to mark or unmark the selected item
	Top	Move to the top of the list of hits
	Page Up	Move up the list one page
	Up	Move one term up the list
	View Results	Display the full details about the highlighted entry
	Down	Move one term down the list
	Page Down	Move down the list one page
	Bottom	Move to the bottom of the list
	Help	Access to the electronic Help screens

Icons on the structure drawing screen

New	Start a new structure
Save	Save the current structure
List File	List the available structures
Print	Print the current structure
Undo	Undo the last action
Cut	Cut the selected area to the clipboard
Copy	Copy the selected area to the clipboard
Paste	Paste clipboard contents into the current structure
Shortcut	Select a shortcut
Variable	Select a variable
Query Verify	Verify query attributes on a node or bond
Preferences	Structure drawing and chemical preferences
Desktop	Set desktop preferences
Fuse	Fuse two fragments together
Center	Center the structure in the drawing window
Carbons	Change display of carbon atoms (dot, C or angle)
Reaction	Toggle display of reaction data
Start Search	Start search for current structure
Save Query	Save a query file
Open Query	Open a query file
Help	Show structure drawing help

The drawing palette

 Pencil Tool

Ring Tool

Chain Tool

Eraser Tool

Selection Tool

Lasso Tool

Text Tool

Set position of this toolbar

Reaction Arrow Tool *not used in this application*

Reaction Role Tool *not used in this application*

Reaction Site Tool *not used in this application*

Reaction Mapping Tool *not used in this application*

Icons at top of Entry Display

 Close Entry

Print Entry

Mark/Unmark

Copy

Diagram on/off

Export diagram

Previous hit

Next hit

ABBREVIATIONS IN THE MONOGRAPHS

abs config.	absolute configuration
alc, alcoh	alcohol, alcoholic
compd/cpd	compound
compn	composition
cryst	crystalline or crystal
crystn	crystallization
dec/decomp	decompose(s)/decomposition
determn	determination
dil	dilute
esp	especially
evapn	evaporation
im	intramuscular
inorg	inorganic
insol	insoluble
ip	intraperitoneal
isoln	isolation
iv	intravenous
max	maximum
mfg, manuf	manufacture
min	minimum
misc	miscible
mixt	mixture
org	organic
ppt/pptd	precipitate/precipitated
prepn	preparation
satd	saturated
sc	subcutaneous
sepn	separation
sol	soluble
soln	solution
soly	solubility
suppl	supplement
tech	technical
temp	temperature

INDEX